Functional Interdisciplinary–Transdisciplinary

Therapy (FITT) Manual

Deborah M. Schott

Judy D. Burdett

Beverly J. Cook

Karren S. Ford

Kathleen M. Orban

Venture Publishing, Inc. State College, Pennsylvania

Production Manager: Richard Yocum
Manuscript Editing: Valerie Fowler, Michele L. Barbin
Cover by Echelon Design

Library of Congress Catalogue Card Number 2003110573
ISBN 1-892132-46-X

Acknowledgments

Thanks to our colleagues at Morton Plant North Bay Hospital for their help in testing each of the activities in this manual. We'd also like to thank those individuals who were hospitalized in the Rehabilitation Unit at Morton Plant North Bay Hospital in New Port Richey, Florida, during the first three months of 2000. Without their willing participation, we wouldn't be able to confidently recommend this manual to our peers. We enjoy the encouragement and support of some exceptional associates, including our Director of Rehabilitation Services, Robert Soleo (MS, CCC/SLP), and our Medical Director, Dr. Ramana Amar. They challenged us to look beyond traditional therapy methods for solutions that meet the needs of patients and professionals in an ever-changing healthcare environment.

We also wish to express our deepest gratitude to Fran Soleo, who donated her time and talents to proofread the original version of this manual. Additionally, we wish to acknowledge Joanne Zarrillo, who helped us to begin our journey toward completion of this manual by authoring our written agreement with each other.

Table of Contents

Introduction

What Is Functional Interdisciplinary–Transdisciplinary Therapy (FITT)?

FITT is best described as therapy that targets a variety of rehabilitation goals to improve multiple physical and mental abilities. All therapy activities found in this manual have been developed to accomplish these goals.

Why Should You Use This Manual?

When deciding on the format for this therapy manual, the authors intended to create a resource to benefit both therapists and clients. They placed importance on designing activities that any licensed rehabilitation professional could facilitate with minimal preparation while keeping therapy purposeful and enjoyable for clients.

When Is the Optimum Time To Initiate FITT?

The National Rehabilitation Hospital in Washington, DC, suggested that the continuing reduction in healthcare spending should spur therapists to develop ways to "cut, prune, and retool" existing therapy delivery models. Most providers are finding that one-on-one direct therapy has become impractical, and interdisciplinary team members must attend to the individual needs of patients in group settings. In the vacuum created by staff reductions, collaboration helps to stretch human resources.

Who Should Use These Therapy Activities?

Rehabilitation professionals affected by managed care, Medicare payment reform, and staff consolidation should be able to use this manual with measurable success.

Where Can FITT Be Implemented?

Providers may use FITT wherever it is important to deliver quality care while effectively managing time, cost, and therapeutic outcomes. Delivery of services using these activities may occur in acute rehabilitation, long-term care facilities, or transitional care units.

Which Clients Can Participate in FITT Activities?

Unless otherwise noted, activities are appropriate for patients/clients with hemiplegia, head trauma, Parkinson's disease, hip fracture/replacement, knee replacement, generalized weakness and debilitation, or chronic obstructive pulmonary disease (COPD).

How To Use the FITT Manual

The following table is a reference guide that shows at a glance which activities target which modalities. The activities themselves are separated into individual sections, including

1. Goals

2. Materials/supplies/personnel

3. Preparation

4. Procedure

Each activity also includes an Activity Assessment Skills Checklist. The checklist allows the facilitator to record the successful acquisition of therapy goals targeted for each client/participant. For the purpose of this manual, a facilitator is needed to lead each of the activities. The authors intend that the facilitator be any *licensed* rehabilitation professional—including RPT, RPTA, OTR/L, COTA, SLP, SLPA, and CTRS—and that nonlicensed employees, trained family members, or trained volunteers be used as aides.

The activities lend themselves to a multitude of variations, and therapists are encouraged to modify or to adapt the activities to best suit the needs of their clients. In some instances, alternatives are suggested to increase the difficulty of the tasks or to provide substitutions for materials/supplies.

ACTIVITY	AMBULATION	AUDITORY COMPREHENSION	BALANCE	COGNITION	ENDURANCE	FINE MOTOR SKILLS	HAND-EYE COORDINATION	MEMORY SKILLS	MOBILITY	POSTURE	RANGE OF MOTION	SAFETY	SOCIALIZATION	STRENGTH	TRANSFERS	VISUAL SKILLS
Bags in the Basin			✓	✓			✓		✓				✓			✓
Exerdice		✓	✓			✓		✓			✓		✓	✓		✓
Frisbee Shuffle		✓	✓	✓			✓		✓				✓			
Hat Tricks			✓	✓		✓			✓		✓		✓			✓
Holiday Fishing	✓		✓	✓	✓		✓		✓			✓	✓			
Hot Spot		✓	✓				✓	✓	✓				✓		✓	✓
Rehab Says		✓	✓					✓	✓		✓		✓			✓
Relay Soccer	✓				✓			✓			✓		✓		✓	
Ring the Bell	✓			✓	✓					✓	✓		✓		✓	
Safety Golf			✓				✓	✓				✓	✓			
Sound Cues								✓			✓		✓		✓	✓
Tic-Tac-Go		✓	✓	✓			✓	✓	✓		✓	✓	✓			
Toss-Scotch			✓	✓					✓			✓	✓			✓
Wall Puzzles		✓							✓		✓		✓		✓	
Wheelchair Aerobics			✓								✓		✓	✓		

Bags in the Basin

Goals

1. To improve standing or sitting balance
2. To improve hand-eye coordination
3. To improve depth perception and number recognition
4. To improve mobility of the shoulder, elbow, and wrist
5. To improve thought organization and simple addition skills
6. To improve socialization and cooperation in team play

Materials/Supplies/Personnel

1 facilitator

1 aide (depends on group size)

5 basins or buckets

5 beanbags

1 photocopy of each point page (5 total)

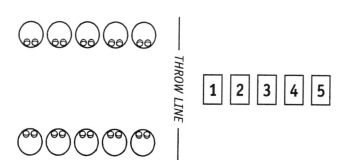

Preparation

1. Seat the clients in two rows, facing each other.
2. Position a point page in each basin so that it stands against the back of the basin and faces the client.
3. Arrange the basins in a single-file line so that each basin and the point page positioned in the basin can be seen easily by the client when seated at the head of the line.
4. Have clients sit or stand at the head of the line of basins to attempt the toss.

Procedure

1. The object of this activity is to earn points individually or as part of a team effort by tossing beanbags into numbered basins.
2. Each client has the opportunity to toss beanbags at any of the five numbered basins.
3. After tossing, points are totaled by the client to practice number recognition and simple addition.
4. The client who takes the first turn will toss until he or she misses a basin, then a client from the opposing team takes a turn. The facilitator keeps a running total of points earned to determine the winning team or individual.

Activity Assessment Skills Checklist for Bags in the Basin

1. To improve standing or sitting balance

   _____ moves from sitting to standing with minimal assistance

   _____ maintains balance while shifting weight forward (while standing)

   _____ maintains balance while leaning forward (while sitting)

2. To improve hand-eye coordination

   _____ maintains forward eye gaze on basins while tossing beanbag

3. (a) To improve depth perception

   _____ lands beanbags in/near basins positioned in a single-file line at progressive distances

   (b) To improve number recognition

   _____ verbally labels the number of the basin into which the beanbag is tossed

   _____ if nonverbal, gazes toward basin indicated when hearing the number

4. To improve mobility of the shoulder, elbow, and wrist

   _____ demonstrates within normal limits/within functional limits (WNL/WFL) wrist flexion and extension

   _____ demonstrates WNL/WFL elbow flexion and extension

   _____ demonstrates adequate motion at the shoulder for underhand toss

5. (a) To improve thought organization

   _____ demonstrates comprehension that the desired objective of the activity is to amass the largest point total

   _____ demonstrates knowledge of turn taking

   (b) To improve simple addition skills

   _____ correctly adds own point total

6. To improve socialization and cooperation in team play

   _____ demonstrates encouragement for his or her teammates

   _____ demonstrates active attention throughout the activity

1

one

2

two

3

three

4

four

5

five

Exerdice

Goals

1. To improve auditory attending
2. To improve standing balance
3. To increase range of motion (ROM)
4. To improve recall of verbal instructions
5. To improve fine motor skills and finger dexterity
6. To encourage socialization in a group activity

Materials/Supplies/Personnel

1 facilitator

1 pair of six-sided dice

1 cup

activity list

Preparation

Seat clients in wheelchairs or standard chairs, facing the facilitator across the table. Engage brakes on wheelchairs.

Procedure

1. Place dice within reach of the first participant in a way that will require him or her to stretch.
2. The client exercises fine motor skills to retrieve the dice from the table.
3. The client places the dice in the cup, shakes the cup, then rolls the dice onto the tabletop.
4. The client or facilitator calls out the number rolled.
5. The facilitator reads the corresponding activity from the list.
6. On each subsequent turn, the client(s) should be given the opportunity to recall the activity/exercise that matches the number on the dice, if it had been rolled previously. This will help to improve memory for information/behavior both heard and observed.
7. Compromised clients may use the table to stabilize balance in standing activities.

Activity Assessment Skills Checklist for Exerdice

1. To improve auditory attending

   _____ demonstrates active attention throughout length of activity

2. To improve standing balance

   _____ moves from sitting to standing with minimal assistance

   _____ maintains balance with/without grasping table's edge while shifting weight forward

3. To increase ROM

   _____ demonstrates full arm extension to reach for dice

   _____ opens fingers prior to grasping the cup

   _____ closes fingers around the cup

   _____ demonstrates active ROM for wrist flexors and extensors

4. To improve recall of verbal instructions

   _____ immediately follows the verbal instructions for each activity

   _____ recalls the activity to be performed upon hearing/seeing the number on subsequent turns

5. To improve fine motor skills and finger dexterity

   _____ uses finger/thumb in pincer grasp to retrieve dice

6. To encourage socialization in a group activity

   _____ interacts with others appropriately

   _____ demonstrates knowledge of turn taking

Exerdice Activities

When the number rolled is	**Clients do this**
2	Kick your right or left leg up 2 times
3	Raise your arms overhead 3 times
4	Shout the numbers 1 through 4
5	Keep your heels on the floor while tapping your toes 5 times
6	With your hands hanging at your sides, roll shoulders forward 6 times
7	Stand up, then clap your hands 7 times
8	Sit and march in place while counting aloud to 8
9	Keep your toes on the floor and lift your heels 9 times
10	Turn head to the right and left alternately, 5 times in each direction
11	Stand and march in place while counting to 11
12	Pat yourself on the head 6 times with your right hand, then 6 times with your left

Frisbee Shuffle

Goals

1. To improve auditory comprehension

2. To improve balance

3. To improve knowledge of ambulation devices

4. To improve hand-eye coordination

5. To improve knee flexion

6. To increase socialization through modified leisure activity

Materials/Supplies/Personnel

1 facilitator

1 aide

1 axillary crutch with pad removed

masking tape

1 Frisbee

paper targets

light weights or bean bags (optional; to place in upside-down Frisbee)

Preparation

1. This activity is especially suited for a long room or hallway.

2. Seat clients facing the Frisbee shuffleboard, composed of the five paper targets arranged in a line approximately 5 feet from the starting line.

3. Place a 12-inch piece of masking tape on the floor for the clients to stand behind.

4. Explain that the object of the activity is to name the ambulation device they currently use, to aim for the paper target with the name of their device printed on it, and to knock the target over with the Frisbee.

Procedure

1. Each client takes several turns by inverting and using the crutch to push the Frisbee toward the paper target with the name of his or her ambulation device on it.

2. Points are scored when the paper target is knocked over.

3. The degree of difficulty may be increased by increasing the distance or the angle between the starting line and the targets or by adding weight to the Frisbee.

Activity Assessment Skills Checklist for Frisbee Shuffle

1. To improve auditory comprehension

    _____ accurately follows verbal instructions

2. To improve balance

    _____ moves from sitting to standing position with minimal assistance

    _____ maintains balance while shifting weight forward with arm extended

    _____ maintains balance while shifting weight from front leg to back leg

3. To improve knowledge of ambulation devices

    _____ verbally names the device used during ambulation

    _____ recognizes name of device on printed target

4. To improve hand-eye coordination

    _____ maintains forward eye gaze on targets while pushing Frisbee with crutch

5. To improve knee flexion

    _____ demonstrates 45–90 degrees of flexion at the knee on the forward leg during lunge

6. To increase socialization through modified leisure activity

    _____ interacts with others appropriately

    _____ demonstrates encouragement of others

ROLLING

WALKER

F O L D

HEMI-WALKER

F O L D

STRAIGHT

CANE

. . . . F O L D . . . .

QUAD-CANE

F
O
L
D

STANDARD

WALKER

F O L D

Hat Tricks

Goals

1. To improve fine motor skills
2. To improve mobility at the wrist, elbow, and finger joints
3. To improve depth perception
4. To improve simple addition skills
5. To improve hand-eye coordination
6. To improve sitting or standing balance
7. To encourage socialization in a group activity

Materials/Supplies/Personnel

1 facilitator or aide for every four clients

1 deck of cards for every four clients

1 hat or container to catch the cards per group

Preparation

1. Seat the clients in a circle around the upside-down hat or upright container into which they will be tossing the cards.
2. Separate the deck of cards into the four suits and give one complete suit to each client.

Procedure

1. Each client will take a turn at tossing all of his or her cards one at a time into the hat/container until the suit is finished.
2. Cards that land in the hat are collected by the client for tabulation. The facilitator chooses the position of the container to allow for assessment of adequate depth perception during card retrieval.
3. While the first client is adding the face value of the cards retrieved from the container, the next client proceeds to toss his or her cards toward the hat. Aces count as 1 point, 2–10 are face value, and all face cards (i.e., kings, queens, jacks) are worth 10 points.
4. Each client takes a turn tossing his or her cards and tabulating his or her results.
5. In the event of a tie, the client who tossed the most cards into the hat will be declared the winner.

Activity Assessment Skills Checklist for Hat Tricks

1. To improve fine motor skills

    _____ uses fingers and thumb to manipulate playing cards

2. To improve mobility at the wrist, elbow, and finger joints

    _____ demonstrates wrist flexion/extension during toss

    _____ demonstrates elbow flexion/extension during toss

    _____ uses adequate finger extension to release cards

3. To improve depth perception

    _____ demonstrates accurate ability to reach and retrieve cards from hat

4. To improve simple addition skills

    _____ demonstrates ability to add numbers

5. To improve hand-eye coordination

    _____ maintains forward eye gaze on hat while tossing cards

6. To improve sitting or standing balance

    _____ moves from sitting to standing position with minimal assistance

    _____ maintains sitting balance while leaning forward

    _____ maintains standing balance while shifting weight forward

7. To encourage socialization in a group activity

    _____ demonstrates knowledge of taking turns

    _____ interacts with others appropriately

Holiday Fishing

Goals

1. To improve standing balance
2. To improve cognition for reality orientation
3. To improve hand-eye coordination
4. To improve upper extremity (UE) and lower extremity (LE) ROM
5. To improve ambulation for short distances
6. To improve sit-to-stand transfers
7. To encourage socialization during a modified leisure activity

Materials/Supplies/Personnel

1 facilitator

aides (depends on group size)

dowel rod

masking tape to mark edge of pond

twine or light rope (24 inches long)

22 paper clips

1 strong magnet

photocopies of month and holiday cards (*Note:* There are no holidays in August. Also, if Easter falls in March, one may change the April holiday to April Fool's Day.)

Preparation

1. Copy the month and holiday cards from this chapter and cut apart, or print by hand onto construction paper.
2. Tie one end of the twine to the dowel rod and the other to the magnet.
3. Attach a paper clip to each holiday and month.
4. Mark the edges of a "pond" on the floor with masking tape. Allow enough room around the outside of the pond for the clients to walk and to gain access to the holiday(s) and month(s) for which they are fishing. Scatter the months and holidays in the pond with the names facing upward.

Procedure

1. Seat the clients around the outside edges of the pond with enough room to walk safely.
2. Each client will take a turn at fishing for either a month or holiday; the second turn will require the client to capture the month or holiday that matches.
3. Clients may need to stand and walk around the outside of the pond to gain access to the month "fish" that matches the holiday "fish."
4. The aide(s) or facilitator may need to supervise for safety during fishing.

Activity Assessment Skills Checklist for Holiday Fishing

1. To improve standing balance

   _____ moves from sitting to standing position with minimal assistance

   _____ maintains adequate balance while leaning toward fish targets with fishing pole

2. To improve cognition for reality orientation

   _____ accurately matches month to holiday

3. To improve hand-eye coordination

   _____ maintains forward eye gaze on paper fish targets while retrieving them with the magnet dangling from a string

4. To improve UE and LE ROM

   _____ demonstrates flexion and extension at the wrist and shoulder during fishing

   _____ demonstrates flexion and extension at the hip and knee during ambulation and transfers

5. To improve ambulation for short distances

   _____ demonstrates adequate use of assistive device while negotiating the walk around the pond

6. To improve sit-to-stand transfers

   _____ demonstrates safe and accurate sequence for moving from sitting to standing and from standing to sitting

7. To encourage socialization during a modified leisure activity

   _____ interacts with others appropriately

   _____ shares knowledge of effective strategies to succeed in capturing a fish with others in the group

JANUARY

NEW YEAR'S DAY

FEBRUARY

VALENTINE'S DAY

MARCH

ST. PATRICK'S DAY

APRIL

EASTER

MAY

MEMORIAL DAY

JUNE

FATHER'S DAY

JULY

INDEPENDENCE
DAY

SEPTEMBER

LABOR DAY

OCTOBER

HALLOWEEN

NOVEMBER

THANKSGIVING

DECEMBER

CHRISTMAS

Hot Spot

Note: Not recommended for patients who are status post hip fracture or hip replacement.

Goals

1. To improve active listening and auditory memory
2. To improve sitting and standing balance
3. To increase mobility and trunk rotation
4. To improve hand-eye coordination in a bimanual task
5. To improve memory for safety precautions
6. To increase socialization through cooperation

Materials/Supplies/Personnel

1 facilitator per 4 participants

1 aide per 4 participants

beach ball (or balloon or bean bag)

music (e.g., tape and tape recorder)

questions list

Preparation

1. Seat clients in a circle with their backs toward the center.
2. Have question list available.
3. Explain the rules of the activity and cue the music to start.

Procedure

1. When the music begins the clients pass the ball around the outside of the circle. Having their backs to the center of the circle will help to promote increased trunk rotation.
2. When the music stops, the client caught holding the ball is required to answer one of the safety questions.
3. Discuss the answers to be sure that everyone recognizes the correct response and is able to verbalize the answer when it is their turn.
4. Activity may be performed with clients in a standing position.

Activity Assessment Skills Checklist for Hot Spot

1. To improve active listening and auditory memory

    _____ demonstrates recognition that activity begins when music starts and that something different occurs when music stops (e.g., begins passing the ball, stops, holds the ball, and waits for the question)

2. To improve sitting or standing balance

    _____ maintains sitting/standing balance during trunk rotation

3. To increase mobility and trunk rotation

    _____ demonstrates adequate reach with both UE alternately toward right and left combined with trunk rotation to right and left

4. To improve hand-eye coordination in a bimanual task

    _____ maintains gaze on ball or balloon during passing and receiving with both hands

5. To improve memory for safety precautions

    _____ provides accurate answers to safety questions

6. To increase socialization through cooperation

    _____ interacts with others appropriately

    _____ demonstrates encouragement of other participants

Safety Questions

1. Is thick pile carpeting the safest surface to walk on?

2. Is "moving the footrests" the first thing you must remember to do before attempting to exit your wheelchair?

3. Will scooting your buttocks to the edge of the chair make standing easier?

4. Are chairs with rolling casters as safe as chairs without?

5. Is a car with bucket seats the easiest sort of car in which to travel?

6. Are you safe to walk without your walker if you are only walking inside your home?

7. Would it be better to firmly grasp the therapist instead of pushing up from the bed?

8. Are ceramic-tiled floors without scatter rugs the safest on which to walk?

9. Is "locking the brakes" the first thing you must remember to do before attempting to exit your wheelchair?

10. Must the backs of your knees be touching the chair before it is safe to sit down?

11. Is a low, soft couch the safest seat?

12. Is it important to use your walker even when going short distances?

Rehab Says

Goals

1. To improve active listening
2. To improve balance
3. To improve mobility
4. To improve UE and LE ROM
5. To encourage socialization in a group activity

Materials/Supplies/Personnel

1 facilitator

1 aide

game list

Preparation

1. Seat clients in chairs or wheelchairs facing the facilitator. Engage brakes on wheelchairs.
2. Be sure the facilitator can be seen and heard easily by all participants.

Procedure

1. The facilitator explains the basic rules borrowed from "Simon Says" (i.e., Do only those instructions that begin with the phrase "Rehab says." Do nothing unless Rehab says to do it).
2. The facilitator calls out an instruction from the Game List and inserts the phrase "Rehab Says" at his or her discretion preceding any of the instructions.

Game List

Stand up	Do 5 ankle pumps
Sit down	Do 5 glute sits
Do a biceps curl	Do 5 quad kicks
Reach overhead	Tap your toes 5 times
Hug yourself	Lift your heels 5 times
Turn head right, then left	Walk forward 5 feet
Pat yourself on the back	Close your eyes while standing
Do large arm circles	Everybody shout, "Rehab is great"
Do small arm circles	Stand without touching your walker

Activity Assessment Skills Checklist for Rehab Says

1. To improve active listening

   _____ makes eye contact with facilitator while facilitator is speaking

2. To improve balance

   _____ requires minimal or stand-by assistance while

       _____ standing (eyes open and closed)

       _____ moving from sitting to standing

       _____ ambulating

3. To improve mobility while

   _____ moving from sitting to standing and from standing to sitting

   _____ ambulating

4. To improve UE and LE ROM

   _____ elbow extension/flexion for biceps curls

   _____ overhead reaching

   _____ hugging

   _____ patting

   _____ arm circles

   _____ ankle pumps

   _____ glute sits

   _____ quad kicks

   _____ toe tapping

   _____ heel lifts

5. To encourage socialization in a group activity

   _____ encourages other group members

Relay Soccer

Goals

1. To improve standing balance and LE ROM

2. To improve mobility at the knee and ankle

3. To improve sit-to-stand transfers

4. To improve eye-foot coordination and depth perception

5. To improve ambulation for short distances

6. To encourage socialization during a group activity

Materials/Supplies/Personnel

1 facilitator

1 or 2 aides (depends on group size)

beach ball

2 chairs without arms

masking tape

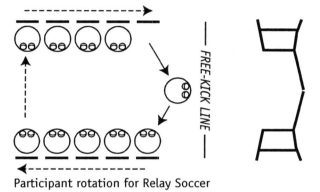

Participant rotation for Relay Soccer

Preparation

1. Seat clients in two equal rows about 5 feet apart facing each other.

2. Place two chairs on their sides on the floor with tops touching so the backs and seats form a "goal net."

3. Put a strip of masking tape a short distance from the chair "net" to act as the free-kick line.

Procedure

1. The facilitator stands at the end of the two rows of clients farthest from the goal and places the beach ball at the feet of the client seated at his or her left, then begins to move toward the goal side of the clients.

2. The client with the ball kicks/passes the ball to the participant directly across from him or her.

3. The clients continue to kick/pass the ball alternating between rows in the direction of the goal.

4. Be sure that each client gets an opportunity to make contact with the ball.

5. The last client to make contact with the ball kicks/passes it to the facilitator who is now between the clients and the goal. The facilitator places the ball on the free-kick line.

6. The client who passed the ball to the facilitator stands, walks to the free-kick line, and attempts to kick the ball into the goal.

7. After the client attempts to score, the remaining clients will stand one at a time with an aide to assist, side-step to the chair on their immediate left, and sit down.

8. The client who takes the free kick will then walk to the chair opposite the one he or she had been sitting in prior to approaching the free-kick line.

9. The facilitator returns to the end of the rows opposite the goal line and begins the activity again. Continue until each client has a chance to score a goal.

Activity Assessment Skills Checklist for Relay Soccer

1. To improve standing balance and LE ROM

   _____ shifts weight without compromising balance while

      _____ moving from sitting to standing

      _____ ambulating

      _____ kicking the ball

      _____ side stepping

2. To improve mobility at the knee and ankle

   _____ adequate joint motion while kicking

3. To improve sit-to-stand transfers

   _____ transfers with less assistance

4. To improve eye-foot coordination and depth perception

   _____ makes contact with the ball during kicking

   _____ maintains forward eye gaze into "net" while striking the ball with foot

   _____ demonstrates adequate force when attempting to score a goal

5. To improve ambulation for short distances

   _____ to the free-kick line

   _____ to the next chair

6. To encourage socialization during a group activity

   _____ encourages other group members

Ring the Bell

Goals

1. To improve ambulation
2. To improve attention and concentration
3. To improve sit-to-stand transfers
4. To improve posture
5. To improve UE ROM
6. To improve memory for new information
7. To improve overall functional mobility
8. To engage in a competitive activity for fun

Materials/Supplies/Personnel

1 facilitator

2 aides (minimum)

2 bells

stopwatch (optional)

timekeeper (optional)

Preparation

1. Seat clients in two parallel rows evenly divided in number.
2. Clients should be seated at least 6 feet apart and facing each other.

Procedure

1. The facilitator stands in a central location, with a bell in each hand, between the two rows of clients.
2. The facilitator assigns consecutive numbers to clients in the first row, starting with the number 1. The opposite row is assigned numbers in the reverse.
3. The facilitator calls out the number 1. Both clients with that number exit their chairs and use their ambulation devices to proceed toward the facilitator in an effort to be the first to ring a bell.
4. The activity continues until each client has a turn to ring the bell.
5. The facilitator has the option to increase the difficulty by positioning the bell at different levels to encourage overhead reaching or knee bending.
6. Increased auditory attention will be facilitated if the numbers are called in random order.
7. Aides provide the stand-by assistance necessary to maintain adequate safety.

Activity Assessment Skills Checklist for Ring the Bell

1. To improve ambulation

   _____ demonstrates adequate balance and gait during ambulation, with or without device, for a distance less than 6 feet

2. To improve attention and concentration

   _____ actively listens to instructions and numbers called out by the facilitator during the activity

3. To improve sit-to-stand transfers

   _____ demonstrates safe sequence while going from sitting to standing prior to grasping their ambulation device

4. To improve posture

   _____ maintains erect spine while reaching for the bell

5. To improve UE ROM

   _____ demonstrates adequate mobility at the shoulder, elbow, and wrist for reaching, grasping, and shaking or swatting the bell

6. To improve memory for new information

   _____ recalls the number that has been assigned and what to do when their number is called

7. To improve overall functional mobility

   _____ demonstrates adequate mobility in UE

   _____ demonstrates adequate mobility in LE

8. To engage in a competitive activity for fun

   _____ actively attempts to be the first to reach the bell

   _____ seeks to improve time taken to complete task (when timekeeper is used)

Safety Golf

Goals

1. To improve hand-eye coordination

2. To improve standing balance

3. To improve sequential memory for items relating to safe sit-to-stand transfers

4. To increase socialization during a modified leisure activity

Materials/Supplies/Personnel

1 facilitator

1 aide

1 standard size posterboard

permanent marker(s)

6 8 ½-by-11–inch file folders

6 large, nonbreakable drinking cups

scotch tape or glue stick

golf balls (hollow plastic practice-type work best)

1 putter per client (or 1 to share among clients)

Preparation

1. Print the *Six Steps To Exit Your Wheelchair* instructions onto the posterboard. Printing should be neat and letters approximately 3 inches high.

2. Cut a circle starting at the folder's edge by tracing around the lip of the cup for each folder.

3. Write one of the italicized words from the chart in block letters above the cutout.

4. Tape or glue a cup to the inside of each manila folder. The folder can then be stood on end forming a tent with the cup as part of its base.

2.

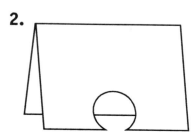

3 and 4.

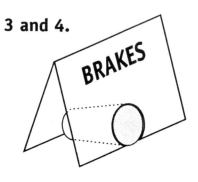

Procedure

1. Place the posterboard with the *Six Steps To Exit Your Wheelchair* in a prominent location that is easily viewed by all participants.

2. Set up the putting green in a small area of a gym or hallway. Arrange the cups in a random fashion to allow for easy viewing as well as easy putting.

3. Position 3 to 6 patients in their wheelchairs so they face the poster and the putting area.

4. Choose a client to begin the game. This client calls out the first step of the wheelchair exiting sequence, then attempts to putt their golf ball into the appropriately marked cup.

5. Each client takes his or her turn by repeating the procedure with the second, third, fourth, fifth, and sixth steps.

Six Steps To Exit Your Wheelchair

1. Apply your *brakes.*

2. Move the *footrests* to the sides of the chair.

3. Place your hands on the *arms* of the chair.

4. *Scoot* your buttocks to the edge of your seat.

5. Place your *feet* on the floor as instructed.

6. *Stand* and grasp your walking device.

Activity Assessment Skills Checklist for Safety Golf

1. To improve hand-eye coordination

   _____ transfers gaze from ball to cup while striking the ball with the club

2. To improve standing balance

   _____ shifts weight side-to-side while putting ball toward cup

3. To improve sequential memory for items related to safe sit-to-stand transfers

   _____ verbalizes or recognizes the correct six steps in the sequence to exit a wheelchair

4. To increase socialization during a modified leisure activity

   _____ encourages other group members

Sound Cues

Goals

1. To improve auditory attention and discrimination

2. To improve reading comprehension and memory

3. To improve auditory memory

4. To improve sit-to-stand transfers

5. To improve UE and LE ROM

6. To encourage socialization through group activity

Materials/Supplies/Personnel

1 facilitator	posterboard
1 aide (if tape recording is not used)	glue stick
photocopies of sound cue squares (1 each)	tape recorder (optional)

Preparation

1. Copy the sound cue squares printed on the following pages and glue onto posterboard as follows:

WHISTLE	Shout first name
COUGH	Lift arms overhead
APPLAUSE	Stand and bow
BELL	March in place (5 steps while seated)
HUMMING	Hug yourself
LAUGH	Flap arms like a bird
"HELLO"	Wave good-bye
PARTY HORN	Kick both legs up

2. Place the posterboard within easy reading distance from the group.

Procedure

1. Instruct clients to listen carefully while a sound is produced by the aide or the facilitator outside the visual range of the participants.

2. Each client will be expected to read the sound cue board to discover which action is to be performed and respond with the correct action.

3. The sounds may be produced in random or sequential order at the discretion of facilitator.

4. To increase the difficulty, the facilitator may produce the sounds in succession with increasing speed or may remove the sound cue board so that the clients would then be required to remember which action was specified by each sound.

Activity Assessment Skills Checklist for Sound Cues

1. To improve auditory attention and discrimination

    _____ demonstrates active listening, verbally or nonverbally (e.g., through facial expression) that he or she hears and recognizes the various environmental sounds/noises

2. To improve reading comprehension and memory

    _____ finds the written description of the sound and performs the activity specified

3. To improve auditory memory

    _____ demonstrates memory for sound and corresponding activity without checking the sound cue board

4. To improve sit-to-stand transfers

    _____ requires minimal assistance to stand and bow

5. To improve UE and LE ROM

    Demonstrates mobility/joint extension and flexion at the

    _____ shoulder

    _____ elbow

    _____ wrist

    _____ hip

    _____ knee

6. To encourage socialization through group activity

    _____ interacts with others appropriately

    _____ encourages other group members

WHISTLE

COUGH

Shout first name

Lift arms overhead

APPLAUSE

BELL

Stand and bow

March in place

5 steps while seated

HUMMING

LAUGH

Hug yourself

Flap arms like a bird

"HELLO"

PARTY HORN

Wave good-bye

Kick both legs up

Tic-Tac-Go

Goals

1. To improve auditory comprehension for yes/no questions

2. To improve sit-to-stand transfers and standing balance

3. To improve memory for safety

4. To improve hand-eye coordination and visual scanning

5. To improve reasoning and problem solving

6. To improve UE ROM

7. To increase socialization through modified leisure activity in team competition

Materials/Supplies/Personnel

1 facilitator	large, sturdy table
1 aide	photocopies of Xs and Os (6 each)
masking tape	additional safety questions (optional)

Preparation

1. Use masking tape to create a large, standard tic-tac-toe board on the top of the table. To increase the level of difficulty for this activity, set up the tic-tac-toe board on the floor to incorporate bending and reaching.

2. Divide the clients into 2 teams of up to 3 players each.

3. Give one team of clients the 6 Xs and the other team the 6 Os.

4. Each client should be holding an X or an O to begin the activity.

Procedure

1. Seat the clients around the table in standard chairs with armrests.

2. The facilitator chooses a team and a player to begin the game.

3. The facilitator asks the first player one of the safety questions from the list.

4. If the question is answered correctly, he or she may stand and place an X or O on the tic-tac-go board.

5. If the question is answered incorrectly, a player from the opposing team has a chance to answer. If correct, he or she would then place his or her X or O on the board. The facilitator provides the correct answer to the group if both teams answer incorrectly.

6. Play alternates between teams until one team successfully places three Xs or Os in a horizontal, vertical, or diagonal row.

7. To play the game a second or third time, you may need to ask additional questions. Consider making a list of questions regarding kitchen safety, community re-entry, or ADL compensatory techniques for the hemiplegic patient.

Safety Questions

1. Is thick pile carpeting the safest surface to walk on?

2. Is "moving the footrests" the first thing you must remember to do before attempting to exit your wheelchair?

3. Will scooting your buttocks to the edge of the chair make standing easier?

4. Are chairs with rolling casters as safe as chairs without?

5. Is a car with bucket seats the easiest sort of car in which to travel?

6. Are you safe to walk without your walker if you are only walking inside your home?

7. Would it be better to firmly grasp the therapist instead of pushing up from the bed?

8. Are ceramic-tiled floors without scatter rugs the safest on which to walk?

9. Is "locking the brakes" the first thing you must remember to do before attempting to exit your wheelchair?

10. Must the backs of your knees be touching the chair before it is safe to sit down?

11. Is a low, soft couch the safest seat?

12. Is it important to use your walker even when going short distances?

Activity Assessment Skills Checklist for Tic-Tac-Go

1. To improve auditory comprehension for yes/no questions

   _____ listens to and answers safety questions with a "yes" or "no" response

2. To improve sit-to-stand transfers and standing balance

   _____ requires minimal assistance to stand up and place an X or O on the board

   _____ requires minimal assistance to stand and bend to place X or O (if board is set on floor)

3. To improve memory for safety

   _____ correctly answers safety questions

4. To improve hand-eye coordination and visual scanning

   _____ finds space and appropriately places X or O on board

5. To improve reasoning and problem solving

   _____ determines logical placement of X or O to "block" an opponent

6. To improve UE ROM

   _____ demonstrates adequate reaching when placing X or O

7. To increase socialization through modified leisure activity in team competition

   _____ recognizes role in team play

   _____ interacts appropriately with team members and other members of the group

   _____ encourages team members

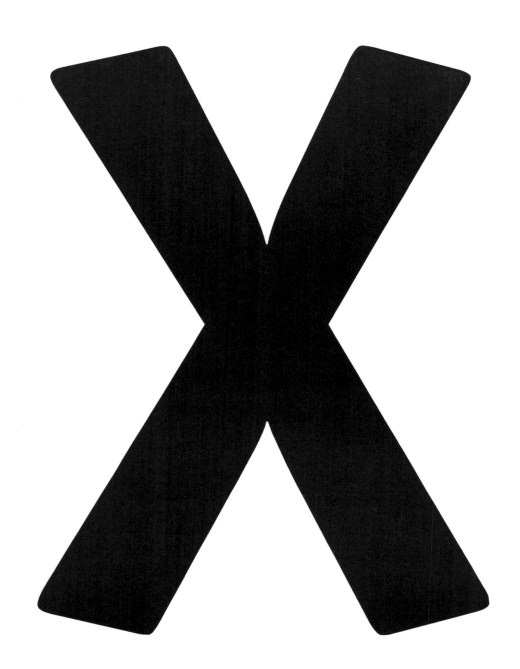

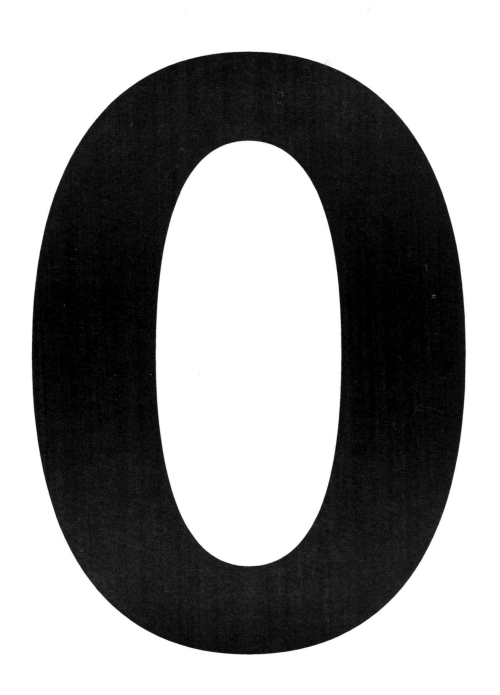

Toss-Scotch

Goals

1. To improve sitting and standing balance

2. To improve hand-eye coordination

3. To improve mobility of the shoulder, elbow, and wrist

4. To improve ambulation safety

5. To encourage socialization through collaboration

Materials/Supplies/Personnel

1 facilitator   masking tape

photocopies of toss-scotch squares (1 each)   bean bag

Preparation

1. Copy each of the pages at the end of this chapter that comprise the toss-scotch board.

2. Place and tape the individual sheets of paper to the floor in the traditional "hopscotch" design as shown.

   A. Linoleum without throw rugs
   B. Ceramic tile
   C. Indoor/outdoor carpet
   D. Low pile carpet
   E. Berber carpet
   F. Shag carpet
   G. Paved sidewalk
   H. Linoleum with throw rugs
   I. Grass, sand, or gravel

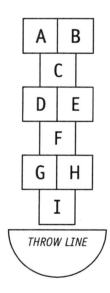

Procedure

1. Each client sits or stands at the base of the toss-scotch board, and takes turns throwing the beanbag.

2. The object of the "toss" is to land the beanbag on the ambulation surface(s) in sequence from the least safe to the most safe (from the bottom to the top of the board).

3. Clients should be encouraged to discuss their options before each turn at tossing the beanbag to gain the consensus of the group.

4. The facilitator is the final judge, instructing as to the relative safety of each surface.

5. Each participant tosses the beanbag until he or she misses the intended target.

Activity Assessment Skills Checklist for Toss Scotch

1. To improve sitting or standing balance

    _____ maintains balance while shifting weight forward

2. To improve hand-eye coordination

    _____ maintains forward gaze on toss-scotch board while throwing beanbag at the intended target

3. To improve mobility of the shoulder, elbow, and wrist

    _____ demonstrates adequate wrist flexion/extension during toss

    _____ demonstrates adequate elbow flexion/extension during toss

    _____ demonstrates adequate motion at the shoulder for underhand toss

4. To improve insight into ambulation safety

    _____ recognizes and/or names walking surfaces ordered according to relative safety for ambulation

5. To encourage socialization through collaboration

    _____ requests and/or receives advice from others prior to tossing beanbag

LINOLEUM

WITHOUT

THROW RUGS

CERAMIC TILE

INDOOR/OUTDOOR CARPET

LOW PILE CARPET

BERBER CARPET

SHAG CARPET

PAVED SIDEWALK

LINOLEUM

WITH THROW RUGS

RUGS

GRASS, SAND, OR GRAVEL

Wall Puzzles

Note: Not recommended for patients who are status post hip fracture or hip replacement.

Goals

1. To improve standing balance during weight shifting activities

2. To increase ability to cross midline (i.e., reach with right hand across chest to left side and reach with left hand across chest to right side)

3. To improve visual perception and left/right discrimination

4. To increase mobility at the shoulder, elbow, hip, and knee

5. To increase UE ROM

6. To improve cognition for problem solving

7. To increase socialization through collaboration

Materials/Supplies/Personnel

1 facilitator

1 aide (depends on group size)

copies of figure outline (1 of each part)

masking tape

Preparation

1. Copy each page of the figure.

2. This activity works best with small groups of 3 or 4 clients each.

3. Distribute the figure by giving several pages to each client until all the pages are distributed.

4. Each of the figure pages represents a separate piece of the large wall-sized puzzle.

Procedure

1. Clients take turns taping their puzzle piece(s) on the wall in an attempt to complete the puzzle. When the puzzle is complete they should have an outline of a person facing them. Clients will need to communicate and to share information with each other to correctly assemble this life-size wall mural.

2. During the assembly phase, clients will be standing, bending, reaching, and communicating while visually assessing their progress.

Activity Assessment Skills Checklist for Wall Puzzles

1. To improve standing balance during weight shifting activities

   _____ forward

   _____ right

   _____ left

   _____ back to neutral

2. To increase the ability to cross midline

   _____ demonstrates reach or total body shift to the right and left when placing puzzle pieces

3. To improve visual perception and left/right discrimination

   _____ recognizes left versus right hand puzzle pieces

   _____ recognizes left versus right foot puzzle pieces

   _____ recognizes and/or names silhouette body parts

   | _____ head | _____ arms | _____ chest | _____ neck |
   | _____ hands | _____ feet | _____ legs | _____ hips/abdomen |

4. To increase mobility at the

   _____ shoulder (for overhead reaching)

   _____ elbow (for forward reaching)

   _____ hip (for forward bending)

   _____ knee (for flexion/extension)

5. To increase UE ROM

   _____ overhead reaching

   _____ forward reaching

6. To improve cognition for problem solving

   _____ recognition/naming body parts

   _____ left/right discrimination/naming

   _____ top/bottom discrimination/naming

   _____ deductive reasoning to recognize which puzzle piece(s) are missing

7. To increase socialization through collaboration

   _____ requests/receives/provides verbal assistance to group members to complete the puzzle

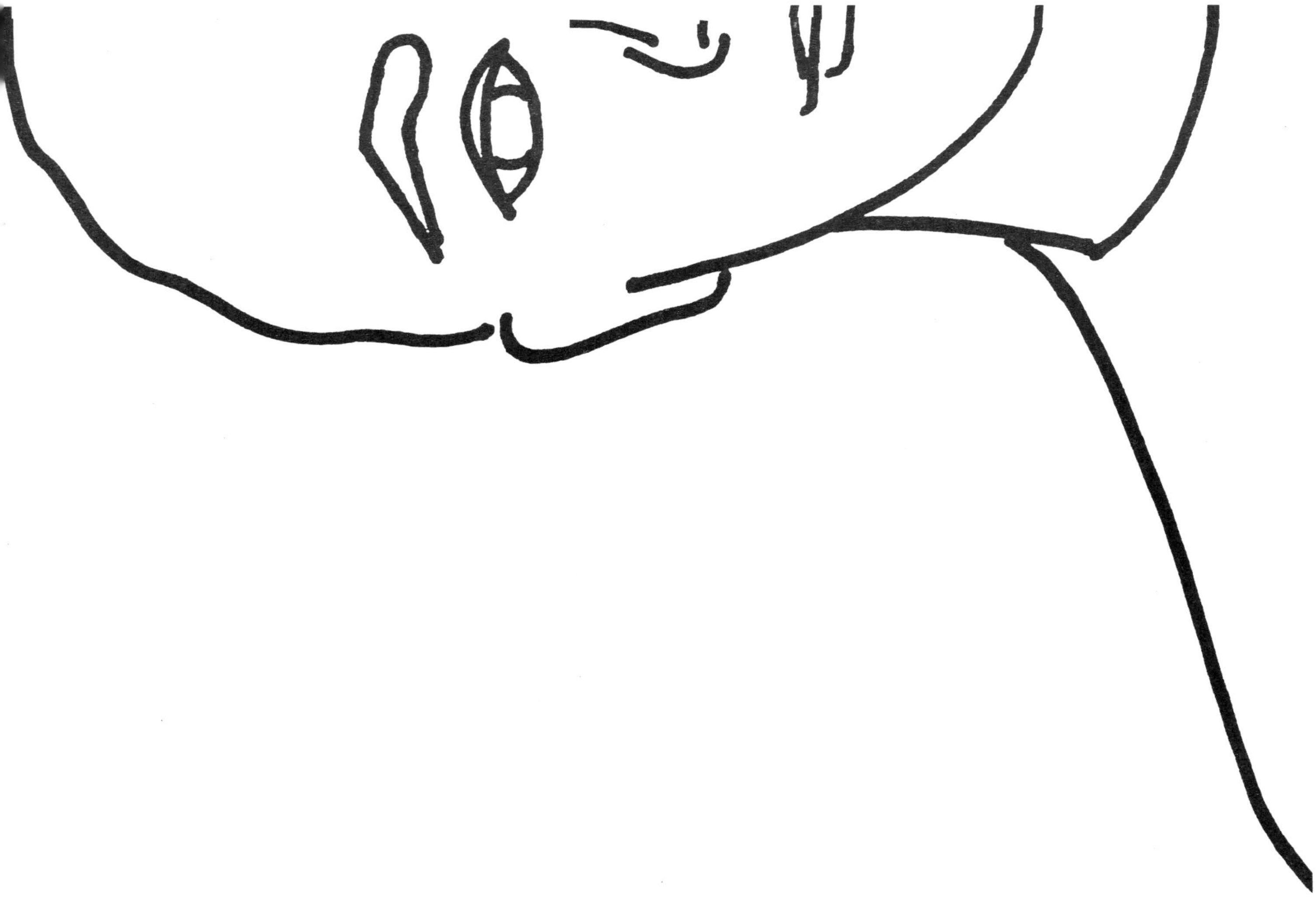

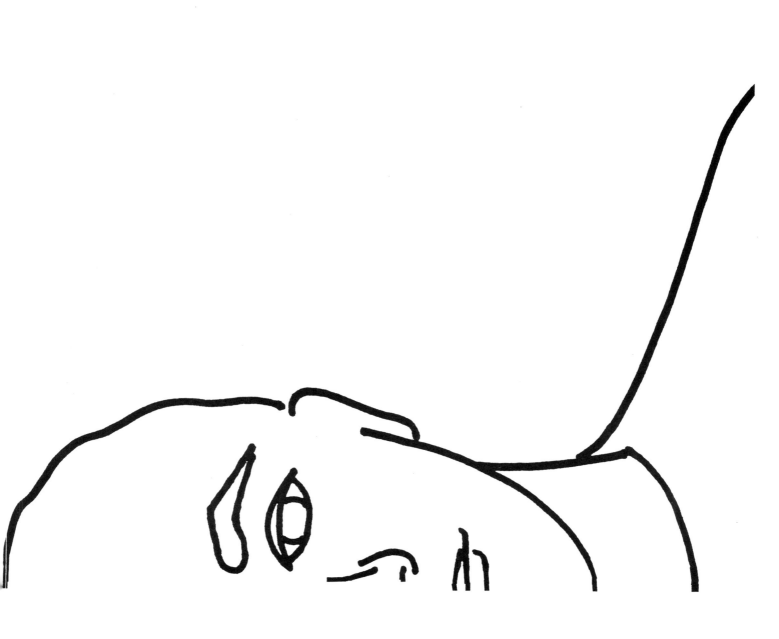

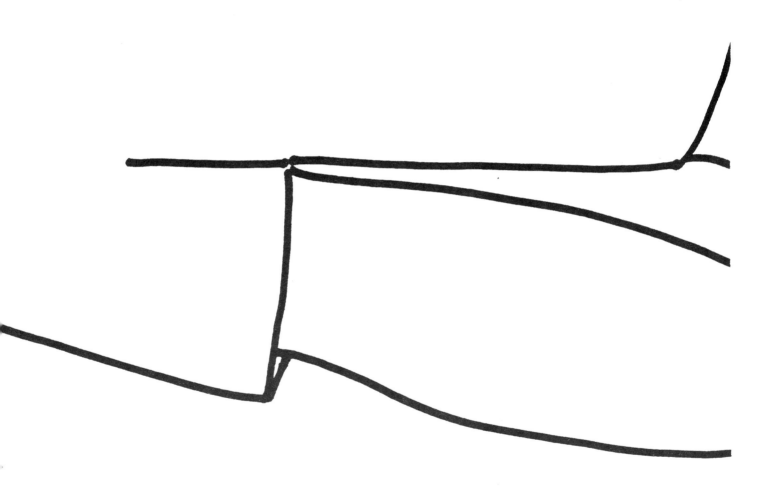

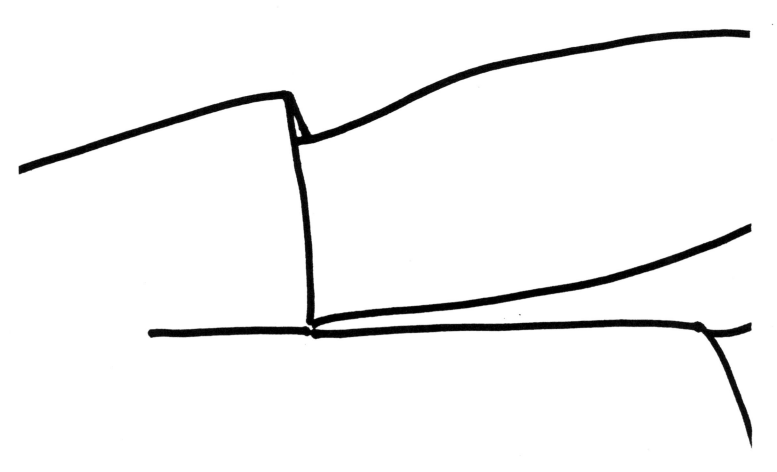

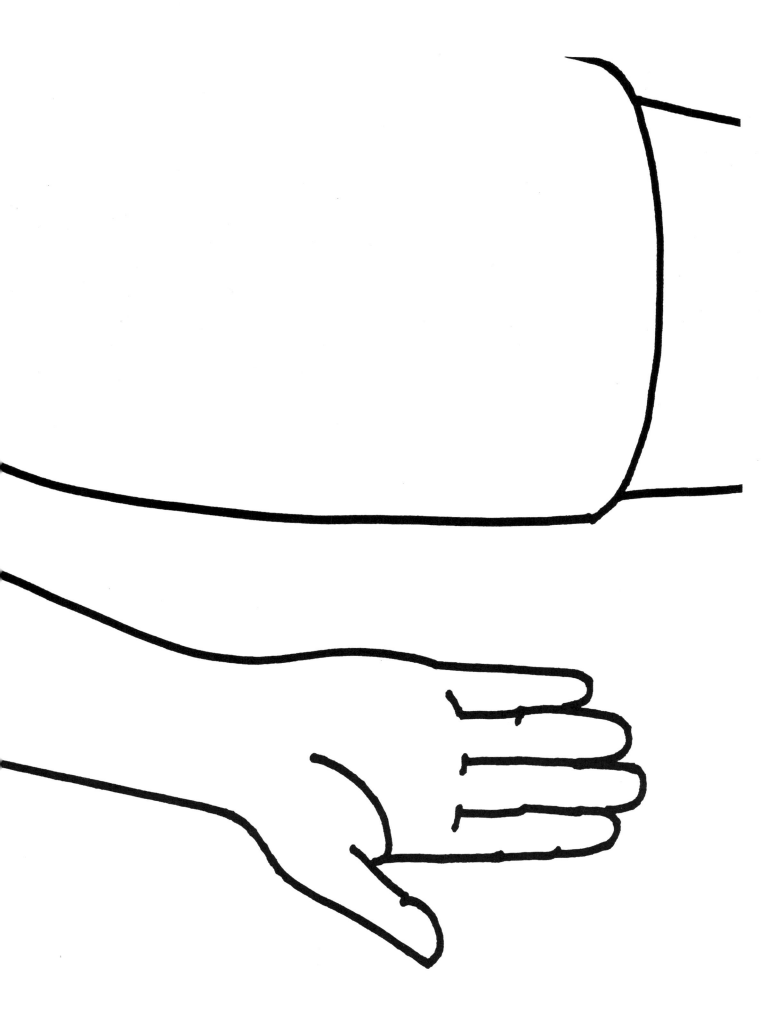

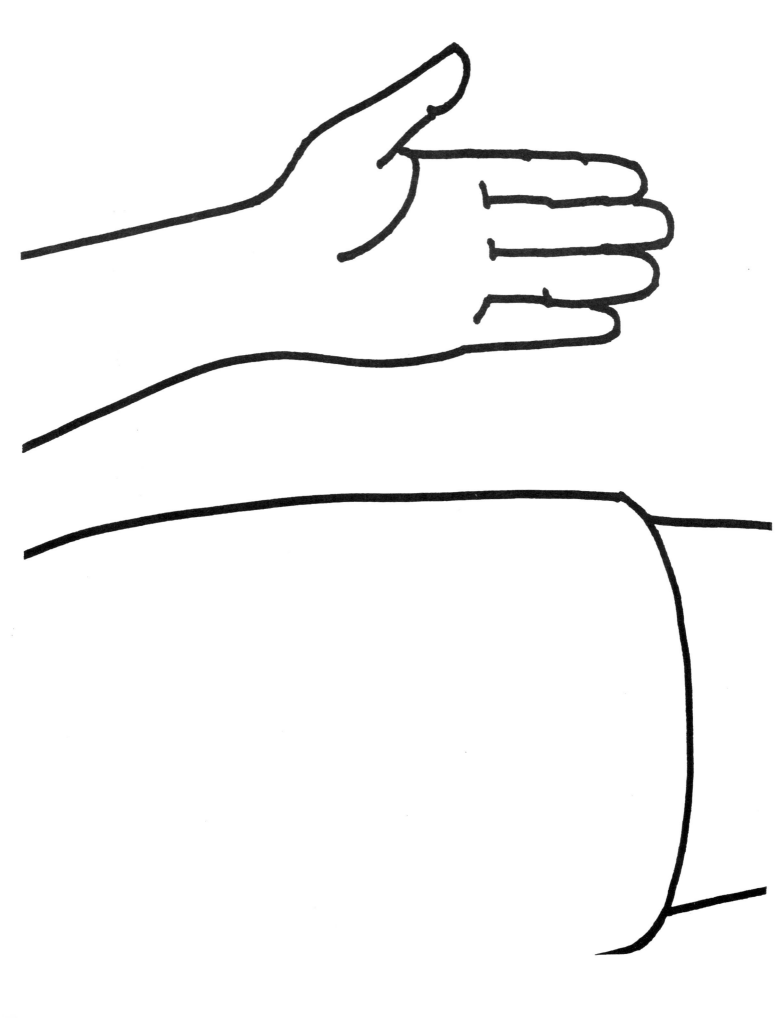

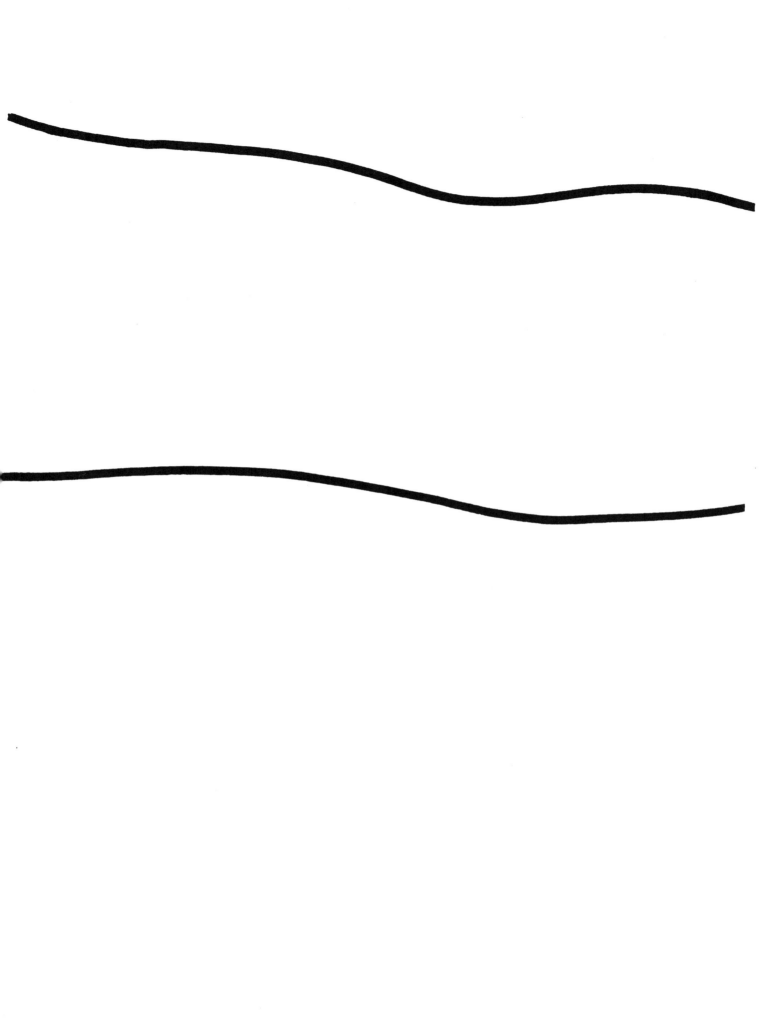

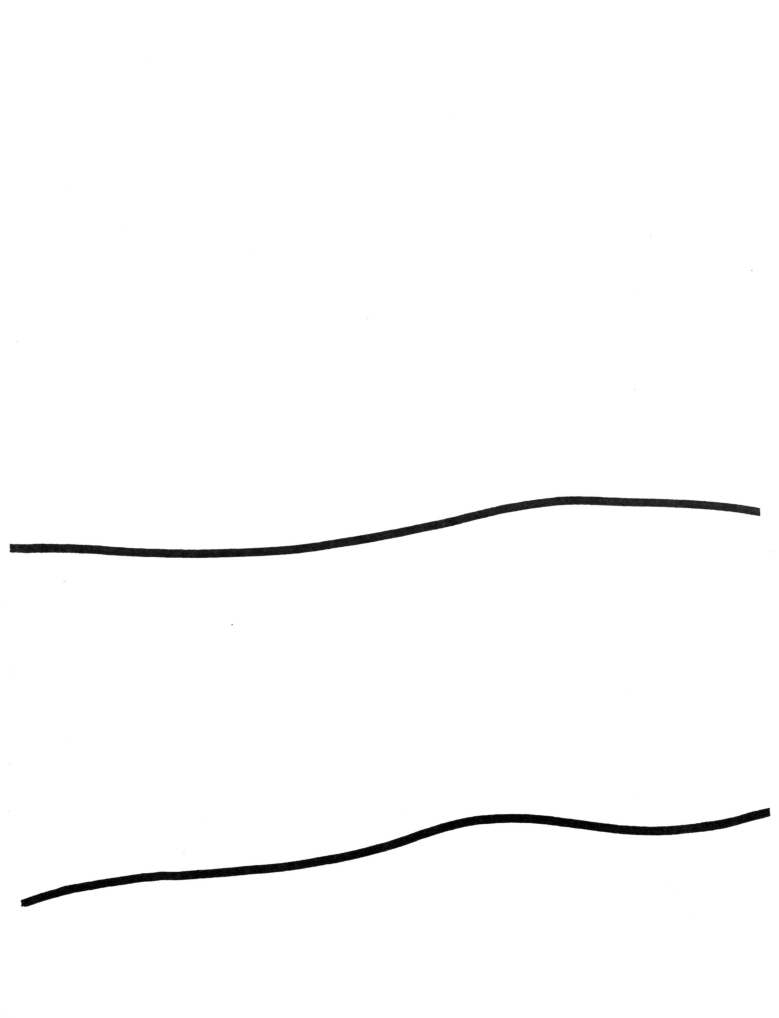

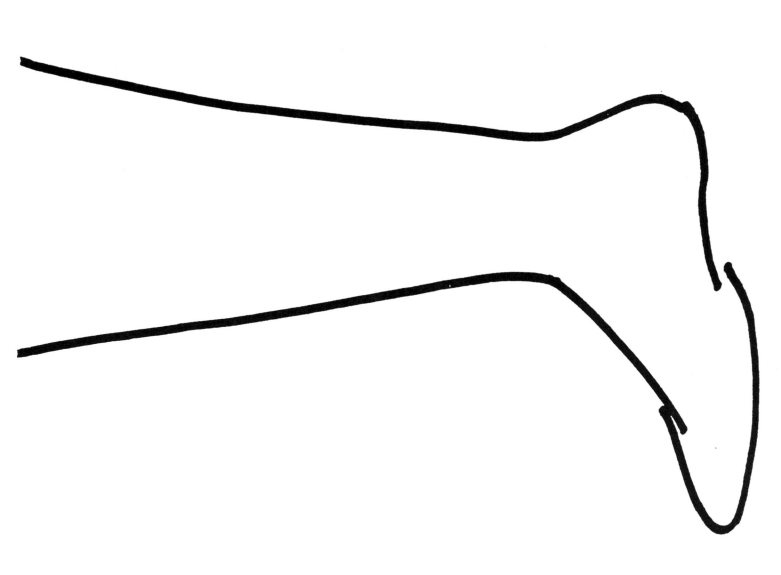

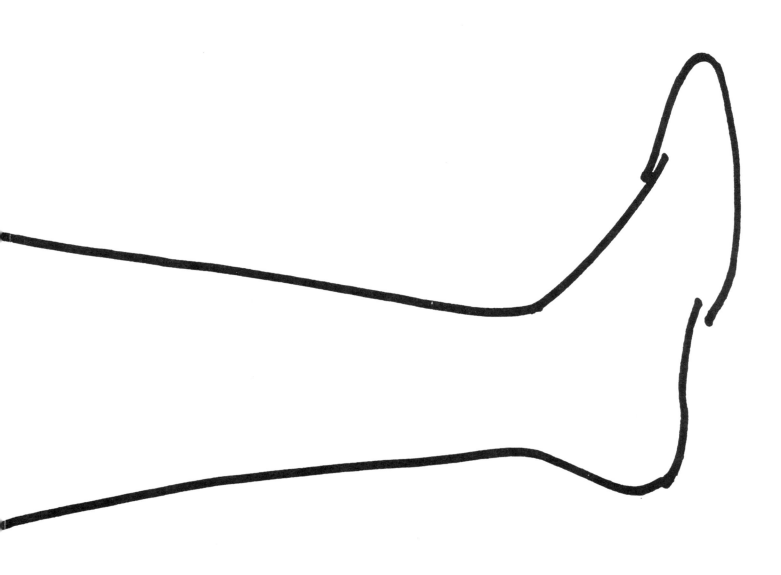

Wheelchair Aerobics

Note: Not recommended for patients who are status post hip replacement or hip fracture.

Goals

1. To improve UE ROM, muscle strength, and joint mobility

2. To improve auditory comprehension

3. To improve sitting balance

4. To encourage social interaction in a group activity

Materials/Supplies/Personnel

1 facilitator

aides (depends on group size)

list of exercises

Preparation

Seat clients in wheelchairs or standard chairs where they can easily see and hear the facilitator. Engage brakes on wheelchairs.

Procedure

The facilitator demonstrates each of the warm-up, workout, and cool-down exercises to the group prior to leading the group in the exercise routines.

Warm-Up Exercises

Relaxed Breathing. Breathe slowly and deeply in through your nose with your mouth closed and out through your mouth with lips pursed. Repeat 2 times.

Head and Neck Stretches. Looking forward, turn head slowly to the right, then turn slowly to the left. Repeat 4 times. Look forward, then tilt head (ear toward shoulder) to the right, then to the left. Repeat 2 times. Beginning with head tilted to the right (ear toward shoulder), roll head forward, chin toward chest, then to the left (ear toward shoulder). Reverse direction. Repeat 2 times.

Shoulder Shrugs. Lift both shoulders toward ears. Relax. Repeat 4 times.

Shoulder Rotation. Begin with arms hanging at sides. Roll right shoulder forward. Repeat 2 times. Roll left shoulder forward. Repeat 2 times. Roll right shoulder backward. Repeat 2 times. Roll left shoulder backward. Repeat 2 times. Roll both shoulders forward 4 times and then backward 4 times.

Lateral Trunk Stretch. Raise left arm overhead. Lean to the right and hold the stretch for 4 seconds. Return to starting position. Raise right arm overhead. Lean to the left and hold the stretch for 4 seconds. Return to the starting position. Alternate left and right stretches, repeating 4 times. Lift both arms straight overhead (as high as possible). Return to the starting position. Repeat 4 times.

End by repeating *Relaxed Breathing.*

Workout Exercises

Biceps Curls. Extend right arm, palm up. Close hand into a fist. Bend your arm at the elbow, bring fist toward chest. Return to start position. Repeat 8 times. Repeat this sequence 8 times on the left and 8 more times with both arms simultaneously.

Salute. Bring hand to forehead in the traditional military salute. Repeat the salute 8 times on the right, 8 times on the left, and 8 times with both arms together.

Turn the Doorknob. Extend right arm forward, elbow should not be flexed. Turn arm and wrist as though turning a doorknob. Turn 8 times. Repeat 8 times with the left arm.

Overhead Reach. Lift both arms overhead. Alternating right and left arms, reach toward the ceiling as though climbing a ladder. Repeat 16 times.

Fists. Hold hands in front of body with elbows bent. Close hands into fists, open hands with fingers spread. Repeat 8 times.

Arm Circles. Extend both arms outward from the shoulders. Keeping arms at shoulder height, circle arms forward 8 times and backward 8 times.

Cross-Country Skiing. With thumbs toward ceiling, swing arms forward and backward alternately. Begin with right arm ahead and left arm behind. Repeat 16 times.

Push and Pull. Raise arms to shoulder height, extended forward. Pull back toward chest 8 times; push forward away from chest 8 times. With arms out to sides, raise hands to shoulders, palms turned up, push up toward ceiling, relax, repeat 8 times. Bring hands under armpits with palms down and elbows bent. Push down toward floor, relax, repeat 8 times.

Hugs. Hug yourself. Turn trunk to the left, hold 4 seconds. Turn trunk to the right, hold 4 seconds. Alternate and repeat 4 times.

Bend-Overs. With feet shoulder-width apart, reach right arm down to touch left foot, reach left arm down to touch right foot. Alternate and repeat 4 times.

Back Pats. Bring right hand up and over right shoulder and bend elbow to pat yourself on the back. Extend right arm overhead and repeat pat 8 times. Repeat entire sequence on the left 8 times.

Chest-Outs. Sit up tall in chair. Pull shoulders back, attempting to squeeze shoulder blades together, hold 4 seconds. Repeat 8 times.

Row the Boat. Extend arms forward at shoulder height, hands clenched and wrists crossed. Pull back while uncrossing wrists, bending at the elbows. Repeat 8 times.

Chest Breathing. Clasp hands behind neck, let elbows fall forward. Breathe in and pull elbows back even with shoulders. Relax and breathe out. Repeat 8 times.

Cool-Down Exercises

Shoulder Rotation (see warm-up exercises)

Shoulder Shrugs (see warm-up exercises)

Head and Neck Stretches (see warm-up exercises)

Straight Arm Stretch. Reach right arm across body with arm extended. Grasp right elbow with left hand. Gently pull arm toward left. Hold for 8 seconds. Repeat sequence on the left. Repeat stretch 2 times with each arm.

Toe Touch. Lean forward with both arms reaching towards toes. Hold for 4 seconds. Slowly return to an upright position, one vertebrae at a time. Returning to the sitting position should take at least 8 seconds.

Hugs (see workout exercises)

Activity Assessment Skills Checklist for Wheelchair Aerobics

Note: This Activity Assessment Skills Checklist only evaluates the activities in the workout portion of the aerobic exercises.

1. To improve UE ROM, muscle strength, and joint mobility

   _____ during the biceps curls exercise, demonstrates adequate ROM during finger flexion, elbow flexion, and extension

   _____ during the salute exercise, demonstrates adequate shoulder abduction, elbow flexion, and extension

   _____ during the turn the doorknob exercise, demonstrates adequate shoulder flexion, forearm pronation, and supination

   _____ during the overhead reach exercise, demonstrates adequate flexion and extension at the fingers, elbows, and shoulders

   _____ during the fists exercise, demonstrates adequate flexion, extension, adduction, and abduction of the fingers

   _____ during the arm circles exercise, demonstrates adequate abduction and internal and external rotation of the shoulder

   _____ during the cross-country skiing exercise, demonstrates adequate shoulder flexion and extension

   _____ during the push-and-pull exercise, demonstrates adequate flexion and extension at the shoulder and the elbow and retraction and protraction at the shoulder

   _____ during the hugs exercise, demonstrates adequate elbow flexion and extension, wrist extension, and shoulder depression

   _____ during the bend-overs exercise, demonstrates adequate shoulder adduction and trunk rotation

   _____ during the back pats exercise, demonstrates adequate flexion at the shoulder, elbow, and wrist; and wrist extension

   _____ during the chest-outs exercise, demonstrates adequate shoulder retraction

   _____ during the row the boat exercise, demonstrates adequate shoulder flexion, adduction, and retraction; elbow flexion and extension; and finger flexion

   _____ during the chest breathing exercise, demonstrates adequate shoulder abduction, adduction, and retraction and elbow flexion.

2. To improve auditory comprehension

   _____ follows the verbal instructions of the facilitator without physical prompting

3. To improve sitting balance

   _____ performs exercises without trunk support while seated in standard chair or wheelchair with armrests removed

4. To encourage social interaction in a group activity

   _____ encourages other group members

About the Authors

Deborah M. Schott (MA, CCC/SLP) graduated from West Virginia University in 1978 with a Bachelor of Science degree in Speech Pathology and Audiology and from Kent State University in 1979 with a Master of Arts degree in Speech Pathology. She has provided speech-language pathology services in a variety of settings, including home health, public schools, skilled nursing facilities, outpatient clinics, acute hospitals, and acute rehabilitation units. She currently provides therapy services to children and adults in Spring Hill, Florida.

Judy Dayton Burdett (MEd, CTRS) graduated in 1986 with a Bachelor of Science degree in Recreation Administration from Southwest Texas State University and in 1994 with a Master of Education degree in Recreation and Leisure Studies from the University of Georgia where she studied with Dr. John Dattilo. She has worked with adults with mental retardation, cognitive, and/or physical disabilities in settings that include group homes, nursing homes, and hospital-based inpatient rehabilitation. She is currently Coordinator of Therapeutic Recreation Services in the rehabilitation unit of a hospital in New Port Richey, Florida.

Beverly J. Cook (CNA, CRA) became a Certified Nursing Assistant in 1979. She became a Certified Rehabilitation Aide and Team Leader for rehabilitation aides in 1983. In 1993, she was appointed Rehabilitation Aide Coordinator and became Patient Care Coordinator in 1997. She has worked with children and adults in skilled nursing facilities and with adults in acute hospitals, inpatient rehabilitation units, and outpatient rehabilitation departments. She was recently promoted to Operations Coordinator of a 20-bed acute rehabilitation unit in New Port Richey, Florida.

Karren S. Ford (BS, PTA) graduated from Western Michigan University in 1970 with a teaching degree in Physical Education. She returned to Kellogg Community College and earned an Associate's degree as a Physical Therapist Assistant in 1991. She has been employed since 1979 in physical therapy departments, serving outpatients, acute inpatients, subacute patients, acute rehabilitation patients, and patients in aquatic therapy programs. She currently provides physical therapy services to acute hospital and rehabilitation patients in New Port Richey, Florida.

Kathleen M. Orban (MS, OTR/L) received her Bachelor of Fine Arts degree from the University of Notre Dame in 1980 and Master of Science degree in Occupational Therapy from Western Michigan University in 1988. She has worked with the geriatric population in a variety of settings, including skilled nursing facilities, subacute facilities, adult living facilities, and camps. She currently serves as the Occupational Therapy Coordinator for acute hospital and rehabilitation patients in New Port Richey, Florida.

Other Books by Venture Publishing

The Leisure Diagnostic Battery: Users Manual and Sample Forms
by Peter A. Witt and Gary Ellis

Leisure Education I: A Manual of Activities and Resources, Second Edition
by Norma J. Stumbo

Leisure Education II: More Activities and Resources, Second Edition
by Norma J. Stumbo

Leisure Education III: More Goal-Oriented Activities
by Norma J. Stumbo

Leisure Education IV: Activities for Individuals with Substance Addictions
by Norma J. Stumbo

Leisure Education Program Planning: A Systematic Approach, Second Edition
by John Dattilo

Leisure Education Specific Programs
by John Dattilo

Leisure in Your Life: An Exploration, Sixth Edition
by Geoffrey Godbey

Leisure Services in Canada: An Introduction, Second Edition
by Mark S. Searle and Russell E. Brayley

Leisure Studies: Prospects for the Twenty-First Century
edited by Edgar L. Jackson and Thomas L. Burton

The Lifestory Re-Play Circle: A Manual of Activities and Techniques
by Rosilyn Wilder

Models of Change in Municipal Parks and Recreation: A Book of Innovative Case Studies
edited by Mark E. Havitz

More Than a Game: A New Focus on Senior Activity Services
by Brenda Corbett

Nature and the Human Spirit: Toward an Expanded Land Management Ethic
edited by B. L. Driver, Daniel Dustin, Tony Baltic, Gary Elsner, and George Peterson

The Organizational Basis of Leisure Participation: A Motivational Exploration
by Robert A. Stebbins

Outdoor Recreation Management: Theory and Application, Third Edition
by Alan Jubenville and Ben Twight

Planning Parks for People, Second Edition
by John Hultsman, Richard L. Cottrell, and Wendy Z. Hultsman

The Process of Recreation Programming Theory and Technique, Third Edition
by Patricia Farrell and Herberta M. Lundegren

Programming for Parks, Recreation, and Leisure Services: A Servant Leadership Approach
by Donald G. DeGraaf, Debra J. Jordan, and Kathy H. DeGraaf

Protocols for Recreation Therapy Programs
edited by Jill Kelland, along with the Recreation Therapy Staff at Alberta Hospital Edmonton

Quality Management: Applications for Therapeutic Recreation
edited by Bob Riley

A Recovery Workbook: The Road Back from Substance Abuse
by April K. Neal and Michael J. Taleff

Recreation and Leisure: Issues in an Era of Change, Third Edition
edited by Thomas Goodale and Peter A. Witt

Recreation Economic Decisions: Comparing Benefits and Costs, Second Edition
by John B. Loomis and Richard G. Walsh

Recreation for Older Adults: Individual and Group Activities
by Judith A. Elliott and Jerold E. Elliott

Recreation Programming and Activities for Older Adults
by Jerold E. Elliott and Judith A. Sorg-Elliott

Reference Manual for Writing Rehabilitation Therapy Treatment Plans
by Penny Hogberg and Mary Johnson

Research in Therapeutic Recreation: Concepts and Methods
edited by Marjorie J. Malkin and Christine Z. Howe

Simple Expressions: Creative and Therapeutic Arts for the Elderly in Long-Term Care Facilities
by Vicki Parsons

A Social History of Leisure Since 1600
by Gary Cross

A Social Psychology of Leisure
by Roger C. Mannell and Douglas A. Kleiber

Special Events and Festivals: How to Organize, Plan, and Implement
by Angie Prosser and Ashli Rutledge

Steps to Successful Programming: A Student Handbook to Accompany Programming for Parks, Recreation, and Leisure Services
by Donald G. DeGraaf, Debra J. Jordan, and Kathy H. DeGraaf

Stretch Your Mind and Body: Tai Chi as an Adaptive Activity
by Duane A. Crider and William R. Klinger

Therapeutic Activity Intervention with the Elderly: Foundations and Practices
by Barbara A. Hawkins, Marti E. May, and Nancy Brattain Rogers

Therapeutic Recreation and the Nature of Disabilities
by Kenneth E. Mobily and Richard D. MacNeil

Therapeutic Recreation: Cases and Exercises, Second Edition
by Barbara C. Wilhite and M. Jean Keller

Therapeutic Recreation in Health Promotion and Rehabilitation
by John Shank and Catherine Coyle

Therapeutic Recreation in the Nursing Home
by Linda Buettner and Shelley L. Martin

Therapeutic Recreation Protocol for Treatment of Substance Addictions
by Rozanne W. Faulkner

Tourism and Society: A Guide to Problems and Issues
by Robert W. Wyllie

A Training Manual for Americans with Disabilities Act Compliance in Parks and Recreation Settings
by Carol Stensrud

Venture Publishing, Inc.
1999 Cato Avenue
State College, PA 16801
Phone: (814) 234-4561
Fax: (814) 234-1651

DATE DUE

MAR 0 8 2008			
APR 1 2 2008			

GAYLORD · · · PRINTED IN U.S.A.